MY MIGRAINE BREAKTHROUGH

MY MIGRAINE BREAKTHROUGH

How I Journeyed out of the Darkness of My Migraines into the Light of a Reclaimed Life

Lee Canter

Forward by David D. Clarke MD

ISBN Paperback: 979-8-9862758-0-2
ISBN Electronic: 979-8-9862758-1-9

Library of Congress Control Number: 2022910729

Portions of this book are works of nonfiction. Certain names and identifying characteristics have been changed.

Printed in the United States of America.

My Migraine Breakthrough
California, United States

www.MyMigraineBreakthrough.org

MEDICAL DISCLAIMER

All content in this memoir is my recollection of what I learned and how I used *The Mind-Body Syndrome* (TMS) treatment approach to help me recover from migraines.

Under no circumstances should any of the content be used as a substitute for professional medical advice, medical diagnosis, treatment or therapy.

Accordingly, for any reason, before taking any actions based upon such information, I encourage the reader to consult with appropriate medical professionals.

THE USE OR RELIANCE OF ANY INFORMATION CONTAINED IN THIS MEMOIR IS SOLELY AT THE READER'S RISK.

TABLE OF CONTENTS

MY MIGRAINE BREAKTHROUGH

FOREWORD

In 1982, while in training at Harbor/UCLA medical center, I met a patient who suffered severe symptoms that had no explanation in organ disease or structural damage. Diagnostic tests were normal, and the cause of her illness was a mystery. In this respect, her condition closely resembled the terrible migraines suffered for years by Lee Canter. Like most physicians, I had no idea how to diagnose or treat my patient even though I was in the 8th year of my formal training. Fortunately, I had heard, vaguely, of psychiatrist Harriet Kaplan, MD who had a special interest in this seemingly intractable problem. I didn't expect much, so I was shocked when Dr Kaplan cured my patient. With instruction from her, I began to learn how to care for the large number of patients with this problem that my colleagues and I refer to as Psychophysiologic Disorders (PPD).

Thirty years and over 7000 PPD patients later, I had met a group of colleagues who did this work, and we founded the non-profit Psychophysiologic Disorders Association. Our mission is to provide for healthcare professionals and the public what Dr. Kaplan had provided for me. Lee Canter joined our Board of Directors and has provided thoughtful insight and steadfast wisdom for several years. His book provides the same and fills an important need, so I felt honored when he asked me to write these words.

There are many excellent, evidence-based books on the treatment of PPD (for which Lee uses the less jaw-breaking term of the Mind-Body Syndrome or TMS), but these books are written by healthcare professionals about their patients. Missing from this library is the patient's voice, an account of the subjective experience of suffering, of trying every possible medical treatment, of the understandable skepticism that mere stress could possibly be responsible for real pain, of the difficult work of tracing all the root causes even when they lead back to childhood and finally of the rewarding triumph that relieving pain also brings with it positive change in many other aspects of life.

Lee's account of this journey is clear, concise, unvarnished, honest, moving, and inspiring. Everyone with pain or another physical symptom that is not linked to an organ disease or structural damage or who is not responding to medical treatment as expected can benefit from the guidance provided by Lee's journey from unrelenting suffering to pain relief through self-discovery. It is a journey that should be made available to all afflicted with PPD/TMS. I can only imagine the benefit to my practice if someone had handed me Lee's book in 1982 and said, "Here is the story of 1/3 of the patients you will see for the rest of your career."

David D. Clarke MD
President, Psychophysiologic Disorders Association

Author of *They Can't Find Anything Wrong!* and editor of *Psychophysiologic Disorders: Trauma Informed, Interprofessional Diagnosis and Treatment.*

Portland, OR
May, 2022

INTRODUCTION

My Journey into Darkness

Migraines haunted me from the time I was an adolescent. To my dismay, as I aged their frequency increased until I entered the world of being a "*chronic migraine sufferer.*" My days, weeks, months, and years were filled with pain, nausea, dizziness, fear, and dread. I simply felt my life slipping away.

As my migraines worsened, I began frantically searching the web for doctors and treatments who could possibly offer relief. This led me to seek help from numerous neurologists, some of whom were practicing in leading migraine treatment centers across the country. The treatments I tried ranged from many different medications, Botox, DHE infusions, Transcranial Magnetic Stimulation, and I could go on and on, yet nothing I was prescribed helped. Instead, all I got were uncomfortable side effects and expensive medical bills. At my lowest point, I became medically addicted to the opioids that were prescribed to me and had to go into a detox facility.

I then of course tried alternative treatments as well. Acupuncturists, osteopaths, herbalists, homeopaths, pain therapists were among the mix I tried, all of which failing to create any lasting results.

To be honest, at this point I gave up hope I might ever recover. I was told that, since my mother and son had experienced migraines, I had a hereditary disorder and that I had to learn to live with it. I reached the point where I became afraid to even hope that I might find some new miracle cure. Why? I found hope to be a demon that would kick me in the gut every time another cure failed to deliver. My life had become consumed by my migraines. It was simply the darkest time of my life.

Steps to My Recovery

At my darkest, I found the *Curable* App by pure coincidence. The information on the app was the first step I took in learning about a breakthrough evidence-based mind-body treatment approach for migraines (known by many names but more commonly) the *Mind-Body Syndrome (TMS)* treatment approach for migraines. In the months that followed, I spent most of my time learning more about this innovative approach and through my efforts I was thankfully able to cure my migraines.

The Curable App jump-started my awareness of the TMS approach. From that pivotal event, my recovery consisted of three fundamental steps.

Step One: Learning about the TMS Approach

It was evident to me that if I was going to consider utilizing the TMS treatment model, I had better learn all that I could as soon as possible. *Mr. Google* became my best friend. Day in and day out, whenever my migraine symptoms allowed, you would find me online. I spent my time searching the web for the recent studies that underpinned the basis for this treatment approach. In addition, I began devouring numerous books written by leading medical practitioners of a TMS approach.

In addition I was fortunate to connect with some fellow migraine sufferers who shared their success stories. They described in painful detail debilitating migraines, no real relief from conventional medical treatments, and then finding and utilizing the TMS approach to reclaim their lives.

Finally, I was able to speak with some leading experts in the TMS field with the support of Dr. Dave Clarke, founder of the *Psychophysiologic Disorders Association.*

My research and reading, interviews with fellow migraine sufferers, and discussions with medical experts helped me understand three key topics that were vital to my understanding of the TMS treatment approach:

- The medical evidence that underpins the TMS treatment approach for migraines,
- How chronic migraines can develop, and
- The new neuroscience of migraine pain.

Step Two: Accepting the TMS Diagnosis and Treatment Approach

In learning about the TMS treatment approach, it became clear to me that for it to be effective, I needed to first accept that I had TMS and that the treatment approach would work for me. That meant that I had to work at determining if I met the diagnostic criteria for TMS and that I believed this was the reason for my migraine symptoms. Then, I had to see if I could accept that the TMS treatment approach would work for me. This process took time and effort but was vital for my recovery.

Step Three: Soothing and Healing My Brain and Nervous System

I knew that as much help as I received from reading, listening, and talking, this alone was not going to cure my migraines. I needed to become the "master of my treatment ship" and utilize the TMS treatment strategies I had read and heard so much about. I began to understand I had the opportunity and ability to soothe and heal my brain. This would be instrumental in reclaiming my life from migraines.

Motivation for Writing My Memoir

I wrote this memoir for several reasons. First, I want to summarize for you, the reader, what it took me over a year to learn about the TMS treatment approach. Thus, if this approach is of interest, I can hopefully save you much unnecessary time and effort.

Finally, it is my profound desire that the story of how I journeyed out of the darkness of my migraines to the light of a reclaimed life will give hope to migraine sufferers who have not been helped by conventional medical treatments.

STEP ONE OF MY RECOVERY

I Learned About the TMS Treatment Approach

CHAPTER 1

The Road to Reclaim My Life from Migraines Began in the Most Unexpected Manner

There is no need to rehash all the dark details of my migraine story. The purpose of writing this memoir is to share how I recovered and not to dwell on how sick I was. Therefore, I can aptly summarize my experience with chronic migraines with the following graphic numbers:

7 years practically bedridden
10 doctors
15 medications
3 hospitalizations
2 pain psychologists
6 alternative medicine treatments

Now, without further ado, let's get right to the steps of how I began to recover from my migraines.

On an unfortunately standard migraine-ridden day, I tried to distract myself from the pain I was experiencing by looking at *Facebook*. I soon came upon an ad for a chronic pain app called *Curable*. I was highly skeptical of any ad proclaiming to have an "answer" to chronic pain such as what I was experiencing with my migraines. However, because I was desperate for any treatment that might help me, I previewed the program.

To my surprise, the *Curable* App introduced me to what appeared to be a breakthrough evidence-based treatment model. This model is known by several names *Tension Myositis Syndrome, Psychophysiologic Disorder*, or, the term I most frequently found, *the Mind-Body Syndrome (TMS).* It is based upon recent medical research that has discovered that stressors both in the present and from the past can result in the development of migraine symptoms in many individuals.

I began to think that maybe, just maybe, the cause of my migraines was not due to a chronic illness but rather to the impact on my neurophysiology of stressors experienced throughout my life.

The *Curable* App started my exploration of the TMS treatment model, but I felt I needed to learn much more about how this model could help my migraines. As I continued to explore, I found testimonials from chronic migraine sufferers who had been able to alleviate their symptoms using this TMS approach. Their stories were very convincing and validated what the research studies were telling me: dramatic improvement could be achieved with the TMS model.

I began to think maybe, just maybe, I too could use these strategies and "reclaim my life" from migraines.

Finally, I also found podcasts where I was able to listen to interviews from leading medical professionals who had used this approach with great success with their patients.

I began to think that maybe, just maybe, the traditional treatment approach I had been relying upon was a "dead end" for me. It was time to take a different mind-body road and act.

The Biomedical Treatment Approach for Migraines

Through my research, I came to understand that there were two treatment approaches for migraines: *biomedical* and the *Mind-Body Syndrome.* I found understanding the differences between the two enlightening and, eventually, a "game changer" in my recovery.

To begin with, the treatments my physicians recommended for my migraines were strongly rooted in what is known as a *biomedical* treatment approach. This approach assumes that migraines are simply caused by *physical illness* in the body and generally excludes *psychological, social, or environmental causation.* Treatments focus on interventions to "fix" the problem, be it medications, mechanical devices, or even surgery in extreme cases.

What was fascinating to me was the lack of a definitive understanding in current medical science. There is simply no medical test that can diagnose migraines. Instead, diagnosis is based solely upon the patient's description of their symptoms. There is no clear consensus as to the physical cause of migraines. Speculation abounds that the causes "may be" a central nervous system disorder or "possibly" a hormonal imbalance or "potentially" a genetic disorder or "theoretically" a vascular irregularity.

Obviously, there are countless numbers of individuals who report being significantly helped by current biomedical treatments. There have been advances in treatments, including CGRP drugs, new triptans, neuromodulation devices etc., that are increasing the number of migraine sufferers who are helped.

However, I was stunned to learn that there are an estimated four million chronic migraine sufferers in the United States alone, myself included, who simply have not responded adequately to biomedical treatments.

The Mind-Body Syndrome (TMS) Treatment Approach for Migraines

TMS, as I just stated, is a new evidence-based treatment model which has helped countless migraine sufferers around the world for whom the traditional biomedical model interventions have not been effective.

The forefather of the mind-body approach to treating chronic pain conditions like migraines was Dr. John Sarno MD. He was a Professor of Rehabilitation Medicine primarily treating patients with back pain. After many years of using conventional treatments with limited success, he eventually started to ask about his patients' broader lives, experiences of trauma, stress levels, and personality characteristics. He eventually came to theorize that most chronic back pain, and eventually many chronic conditions, are in fact caused by what is going on in the brain and nervous system rather than by what is going on in the body.

The medical science around chronic pain and other conditions has advanced dramatically in recent years, validating some of Sarno's theories and expanding upon his initial efforts. As I will elaborate upon further as I discuss my recovery, the Mind-Body Syndrome (TMS) treatment approach is based upon both Sarno's theories and recent neuroscience research.

Among the key concepts of this model that I found most useful to understand were the following:

- Anatomical changes in the brain can take place in individuals experiencing emotional neglect or abuse, physical or sexual abuse, and a host of other stressors. These changes result in becoming more reactive to stress.
- As astounding as it sounds, the physiological impact of such stress can increase the probability of developing physical conditions, including anxiety, depression, cardiovascular disease, autoimmune disorders, fibromyalgia, chronic pain disorders, and, the biggest eye opener for me, migraines.
- In addition, there are several other factors that increase one's level of stress which can contribute to developing migraine symptoms.
    - ◇ First is a genetic factor: "hypersensitivity to stress." Highly sensitive people are genetically more sensitive to stressful stimuli.
    - ◇ Second is one's personality characteristics. Individuals who are perfectionist, highly self-critical, or people pleasers tend to put high levels of stress on themselves.
    - ◇ Third is an inability to express negative feelings such as anger, sadness, disappointment etc. Keeping in feelings is another stress builder.
- New research validates that even though there is not an actual physical illness causing the pain and other symptoms, they are *real.* Having symptoms does not mean one is "crazy."
- Of the greatest importance is the fact that the brain is adaptive. Just as it can be "harmed" by past stressors or learn to "overreact" to stress, there are TMS treatment strategies that can "soothe and heal"

> the brain. By using such strategies, individuals can reduce the frequency and severity of their migraines and even cure them once and for all.

Before I go any further, I must state that many of the recent medical science findings this approach is based upon "fly in the face" of the conventional theories of the biomedical model that I had been steeped in throughout my life, meaning I had to take off my blinders to see the light of a new reality of treatment.

It is vital to recognize that breakthrough medical advances such as we are seeing in this model are typically faced with ridicule, then skepticism, and finally accepted as common sense by the medical establishment. Previous examples include germs causing illness, immunotherapy's capability to cure cancer, and antiseptic hand washing reducing infection. These were all once thought absurd!

Who can Benefit from the TMS Treatment Approach?

I quickly learned that the migraine sufferers who got the most positive results in using the TMS treatment approach had many if not all of these characteristics (these will be discussed in greater detail later).

A physician has ruled out that there is a physical issue that would explain migraine symptoms

First off, individuals must rule out a physical issue causing their symptoms, such as a brain tumor or other type of illness. This means they must have a thorough examination by a physician.

The individual was raised in an emotionally or physically stressful environment

Studies tell us that a stressful or traumatic childhood can be an important factor in the development of migraines. The more emotionally or physically challenging childhood experiences individuals encountered the higher the probability of developing migraines.

It is important to note that many migraine sufferers report they felt they had not experienced severe trauma such as physical, sexual, or emotional abuse, but that they experienced a constant level of stress that was the result of having critical, emotionally distant, unstable, or judgmental parents, serious illness in the family, marital discord, not fitting in with the family etc.

The individual is highly sensitive

Many migraine sufferers can be identified as *highly sensitive persons.* What has been discovered is that highly sensitive individuals have increased emotional sensitivity, higher levels of creativity, richer personal relationships, and a greater appreciation for beauty. On the other hand, such individuals have stronger reactivity to both external stimuli—pain, hunger, light, and noise. They are more disturbed than others by stressful situations or feelings of being overwhelmed.

The individual has migraine sufferer personality traits

From the experience of TMS practitioners, it is quite clear that migraineurs with definite personality characteristics can find this treatment approach highly effective. Such characteristics include:

- Having low self-esteem,
- Being a perfectionist,
- Having overly high expectations of yourself,
- Wanting to be good and/or liked,
- Being overly conscientious,
- Being hard on yourself,
- Being anxious and fearful,
- Feeling overly responsible for the well-being or feelings of others, and
- Difficulty expressing negative emotions.

Individual has or has had other potential TMS symptoms

Individuals whose migraines are the result of TMS often have suffered from other symptoms that medical tests indicate do not have an actual physical cause. The more of these symptoms of conditions that individuals have experienced the higher the likelihood their migraines could be a product of TMS. Among the most common symptoms:

- Fibromyalgia,
- Irritable bowel syndrome,
- Chronic back pain,
- Anxiety,
- Depression,
- Insomnia,
- Paresthesia (numbness, tingling, burning in extremities),
- Tinnitus (ringing in the ear), and
- Chronic indigestion.

What is understood is that the more of these characteristics' individuals have, the higher the probability they can be helped by a TMS approach

CHAPTER 2

A New Perspective on Chronic Migraines: How Chronic Migraines Can Develop

One of the first questions that perplexed me and launched the next search on my journey to recovery was as follows: if migraines do not have an identifiable biomedical cause, why did I get them? The answers I found were nothing I had ever contemplated nor could have believed to be true. They became another significant step on my journey to reclaim my life from migraines.

The Impact of a Stressful or Traumatic Childhood

In the quest for the causes of my migraines, I keep bumping up against one that I could not believe applied to me. Little did I know how wrong I was or how much my doubting response to this cause was shared by many other migraine sufferers and all too many medical professionals.

In my research, I found the dramatic effect that *toxic stress* occurring in childhood can have on mental and physical health in adults. Emotionally or physically stressful or traumatic childhood experiences actually can impact the development and severity of migraine symptoms.

Big "T" versus little "t" trauma

Researchers have identified two types of childhood trauma that can impact the development of migraines: big "T" and little "t" traumas. Big "T" traumas are events most thought of when we hear the phrase "childhood trauma", including:

- A mentally ill parent,
- A chronically ill parent or one who died,
- Living in poverty or in a violent neighborhood,
- Severe physical or emotional abuse, and
- Sexual abuse.

The impact of big "T" trauma on migraines was first publicized through the landmark Adverse Childhood Experience (ACE) study. Using data from 17,000 participants, the study was conducted by the *Centers for Disease Control (CDC)* and *Kaiser Permanente.* It demonstrates that having adverse childhood experiences, also known as big "T" traumas, are major risk factors for various illnesses including heart disease, fibromyalgia, irritable bowel syndrome, and, most importantly for me, also migraines.

Little "t" traumas refer to emotionally distressing experiences that don't fall into the big "T" category. Examples of little "t" trauma include:

- Demanding, critical parents,
- Distant, emotionally neglectful parents,
- Marital discord, separation, or divorce,
- Stressful relationships with parents,
- Sibling who is a substance abuser or mentally ill,
- Parent incarcerated,
- Faced medical trauma,
- Faced racism or discrimination,
- Serious or chronic health issues, and

- Constant bullying or harassment from siblings or classmates.

I was surprised to find studies indicating that many migraine sufferers initially have difficulty identifying little "t" trauma in their childhood. When first interviewed, they reported that they "did not perceive their childhood was overly stressful."

But, in further discussions, it becomes clear they experienced a constant level of stress such as from having critical, emotionally distant, unstable or judgmental parents, serious illness in the family, marital discord, etc. that affected them greatly.

TMS specialist Dr. David Schechter MD (a physician who treated me) discusses in his book *Think Away Your Pain* how many of his patients report experiencing several kinds of little "t" trauma. Some report growing up in a "pressure cooker." Though they describe a happy loving childhood, they felt under enormous pressure to be "perfect" children, students, athletes, musicians, etc. They perceived the love they received from their parents was not unconditional but contingent upon them acting in an expected manner. The impact of the underlying emotional stress they felt remained with them as adults.

Many of his patients also reported that they felt like a "*round peg in a square hole.*" They did not quite fit in with their siblings or parents. For example, they might be more emotional, intelligent, creative, or less athletic, outgoing, or religious. Many found these differences hard to reconcile and that led to loneliness and eventual estrangement from their family.

Though big "T" traumas are perceived as more dramatic and more potentially harmful, researchers now conclude that repeated exposure to little "t" traumas can also increase the probability of developing migraines. In one important study, individuals who reported experiencing emotional neglect as children were 50% more likely to experience migraines than those who did not.

How big "T" and little "t" traumas impact the development of migraines

I was stunned to find that the medical profession is just beginning to fully understand the serious long term impact chronic stress and trauma can have on physical and emotional health. A brief overview on this significant issue is as follows.

Trauma and chronic stress in childhood can produce detrimental changes in the brain of a growing child. Childhood adversity alters neural connectivity in the amygdala (the alarm center of the brain), the prefrontal cortex (the decision-making center of the brain), and the hippocampus (where the brain processes emotions and memories).

It is important to note that all of these changes affect an individual's ability to respond to stress.

Growing up with chronic, unpredictable, toxic stress and not knowing when the next stressful event is coming results in a child living in a low-grade, constant state of alertness, fear, hypervigilance—essentially a low-grade state of fight, flight, or freeze.

This heightened stress response leads to increased production of inflammatory chemicals and stress hormones which can produce long-lasting shifts in the genes that oversee the stress response.

The bottom line is that we now understand the physiological changes trauma and chronic stress produce can be a significant factor in individuals developing migraines.

Reading and hearing that childhood stress could be a factor in my developing migraines was a "jaw dropping" insight. "Never in a thousand years" could I conceive that my body and brain could have been deeply affected by such a factor.

To begin with, I must state that not one single medical practitioner who treated me ever once asked me about my childhood nor mentioned that childhood stress or trauma could be any factor in my migraines.

After much doubt, I finally came to realize that my childhood was highly stressful. There is no way I could describe my childhood as happy. Though my physical needs were always taken care of, the same cannot be said for my emotional ones. My mother was an unhappy, angry person. Though she tried her best, her issues put a "dark cloud" of constant emotional neglect and stress over my formative years.

I was anxious and often afraid of my parents' rejection. I felt there was nothing I could do to get their love and that there really must be something "wrong with me." Like the proverbial "fish in water" as a child, I never recognized how stressful and damaging my homelife was not only on my psyche but to my consternation on the development of my migraines.

I have come to see that for me, as noted author Donna Jackson Nakazawa writes in her classic study of childhood stress, *Childhood Disrupted:*

Time does not heal these wounds. One does not just get over something, not even fifty years later…human beings convert traumatic emotional experiences in childhood into organic disease later in life…… your emotional biography becomes your physical biography. And together they write much of the script for how you will live your life and physical health.

Having a Highly Sensitive Makeup

As my exploration into how migraines develop continued, I became aware of how an individual's genetic makeup can play an important role in a way little understood until the last few years. Let me explain.

Many migraine sufferers can be clinically identified as *highly sensitive persons.* This is a term coined by noted researcher and psychologist Elaine Aron, PhD. What has been discovered is that highly sensitive individuals have increased emotional sensitivity, higher levels of creativity, richer personal relationships, and a greater appreciation for beauty.

On the other hand, such individuals have stronger reactivity to stimuli including pain, hunger, light, and noise. They are more disturbed than others by violence, stressful situations, or feelings of being overwhelmed. They may, as a result, make concerted efforts to avoid situations in which such things are likely to occur.

Studies show that between fifteen and twenty percent of the population have the genetic makeup that results in characteristics recognized as highly sensitive.

Being highly sensitive, I learned, is a particularly vexing issue for individuals who experience stressful childhoods. The majority of non-highly sensitive children show a biological indifference to experiences of excessive stress or trauma. The response circuits in their brains are minimally reactive to such events, meaning they are mostly unperturbed by the adversities they confront.

On the other hand, highly sensitive children show an exceptional susceptibility to both negative stressors and trauma, with response circuits highly sensitive to adverse events. As a result, these children often experience higher levels of emotional and physical illness (including migraines) as they grow up.

Put another way, this means that the frequency and severity of migraine symptoms can result from an individual's genetic sensitivity to stress and not an emotional shortcoming.

Reading about the attributes of highly sensitive people, I immediately began to see how they fit me. On one hand, I've always had more difficulty than others handling stressful situations; be it at home or work, when walking down a noisy street, spending a lot of time with family or friends, or being in pain. On the other hand, I became a successful psychotherapist because I was so attuned to the feelings of others, I am very creative (having written a number of books), and I love the beauty in the photographs I produce.

I appeared to be almost a perfect fit. I must admit that, to me, the "negative" attributes (related to handling stress etc.) also resulted in me always feeling that there was "*something wrong with me that should be fixed,*" but that no matter how hard I tried, it couldn't. I found it enlightening to recognize that so many others had the same attributes as

I and that science now has recognized this was the result of genetics and not some personality defect.

Of greater importance to me was that many health professionals and researchers believe that because highly sensitive people are so much more reactive to stress that this could increase their risk for getting migraines.

Difficulty in Expressing Negative Emotions

As discussed earlier, Dr. John Sarno, a founder of the TMS treatment approach, hypothesized that patients had chronic pain because they repressed and could not feel or express negative feelings, especially anger. Again, TMS physicians who came after him built upon his theory, adding that other chronic conditions including migraines could be the result of repressed feelings as well. They also believed other repressed negative feelings such as sadness and inadequacy could also be a culprit in the development of chronic illness.

When I was first exposed to the theories of Dr. Sarno and his followers, I simply couldn't buy it! I knew that many schools of psychological thought accepted the concept of people repressing threatening feelings but never that this could cause chronic pain symptoms. This theory sounded very far-fetched, even to someone like me who has studied psychology and been in therapy. I would soon find out how wrong I was.

This change of mind was the result of conversations I had with several highly respected TMS physicians, including

David Clarke, MD, the co-founder of the *Psychophysiological Disorder Association* and author of *They Can't Find Anything Wrong,* and David Hanscom, MD, author of *Back in Control.* They both shared their clinical experience treating countless numbers of chronic pain patients, including migraine sufferers. Both doctors were struck by how many of their symptoms improved or ended when they were able to express repressed feelings, often from childhood, that they had not recognized or been frightened to face.

Another way I came to understand the effect of repressed emotions is as follows: the brain processes emotions and pain in similar regions of the brain. When individuals are fearful of expressing certain emotions, such as anger, sadness, or fear, the brain perceives such emotions as a danger signal or threat. The more the brain avoids such emotions, the more readily its "danger centers" are triggered. When the brain's danger centers are on guard, they can produce physical symptoms with greater ease and frequency.

The following analogy illustrates the repercussions of not expressing negative feelings:

Imagine your emotions like a river. If that river becomes blocked, the water will become stagnant, build up, and then jam with even more obstructions. Eventually, the river will become toxic, burst its banks, and overflow.

Unfortunately for many migraine sufferers, when the river overflows, the symptoms begin.

I did not fully grasp the effect repressing emotions can have on the development of migraines until I looked in the proverbial mirror at my own journey. Yes, I had migraines throughout my life and at times they were debilitating, but they became severe at a pivotal point in my life, when "*my emotional river began to overflow.*"

This story begins with my childhood challenges of feeling inadequate and unlovable. Inside me was a great deal of anger for how I was treated as a child. Though these feelings lived inside me, I was mostly able to cover them up. I did this by throwing myself into a professional career where I was more successful than I ever thought such an inadequate person could be. My work became my identity.

This all came crashing down when I planned to retire. On the surface, I couldn't wait to put down the responsibility of my career and have more time with my wife, children, grandchildren, and photography. But unfortunately, in my psyche dark clouds were building. As I came closer to stopping work, I was distressed to have the frequency of my migraines increasing to almost daily. Their severity increased too.

I tried every traditional and alternative treatment and, in total desperation, turned to the TMS approach. As I began to use the strategies I learned, I was shocked, dumbfounded, and flabbergasted by the feelings that surfaced.

Without the distraction of my professional identity, the feelings of inadequacy from my childhood that I could never deal with or express reared their dark and ugly heads. I felt worthless and unlovable not having the recognition and accolades that come with being a successful professional. I simply did not feel I could face life.

Getting in touch with and expressing the feelings of inadequacy and anger that formed this "dark side" that lived in me was at first frightening but then quite liberating. I began to see that my migraines, as horrible as they had been, were the lesser of two evils, with the second evil being the feelings I could not acknowledge. Coping with my migraines was an all-consuming distraction from the repressed feelings I wanted to avoid. Thinking back, what I got in touch with was reflected in the words from the classic song "The Way We Were":

> *What's too painful to remember, we simply choose to forget.*

Having Chronic Migraine Personality Traits

The more I researched the TMS treatment approach, the more surprised I was learning about personality characteristics that can contribute to chronic migraines. Children who grow up in stressful or traumatic circumstances often develop particular personality traits to help them cope. Though these traits may be adaptive at the time, they can have long-term detrimental effects as the individual grows up. Among the most common of these traits are the need to be perfectionist, highly self-critical, driven, anxious, fearful, and also needing to be a helpful "people pleaser." The consequences of possessing such traits can add to the stress that impacts the development of migraines.

Perfectionism

> *Perfectionists unconsciously set up standards for themselves they cannot possibly meet; their inevitable failure to live up to them results in living with the frustration and strain that comes with never being "good enough." Such a perspective results in the brain constantly being in a state of fear.*

Almost every chronic migraine sufferer I have spoken with has, to a greater or lesser degree, perfectionist traits. Even if they did not recognize they had such a trait, they acknowledged that they were highly responsible and conscientious. They felt driven to do things perfectly or right as a result of a deep need to demonstrate to themselves and the rest of the world that they are truly a person of value.

Strong inner critic

Another universal trait I heard from migraineurs was that "voice in their head" that seldom stopped "raging" at them. The overwhelming majority, having been subjected to emotional neglect or abuse as children, grew up believing that this had occurred because there was "something wrong" with them.

The result was to grow up being highly self-critical. There is no question that the voice in people's heads, by browbeating them constantly, sends messages that there is something wrong and increases the level of fear the brain experiences.

Serial caretaker

Another pervasive trait is that chronic migraine sufferers tend to be driven to be helpful, often to the extent of sacrificing their own needs. They take more responsibility to care for others than is appropriate and believe they should care for and keep family and friends happy.

This is often the after-effect of their belief that if they were "good" and "helped out" enough, they would get the love and attention they deserved. From a social and interpersonal perspective, it's wonderful to be perceived as a loving caring person. Doing so within reason has definite benefits, but overlooking one's own needs is a recipe for emotional disaster. This is another cause for an increase in the level of fear.

Anxious and fearful

> *Constantly being anxious and fearful of what is coming around the corner keeps the brain in a regular fight-or-flight state of fear, which is a known trigger for migraines.*

The stress of living in a home environment that was unstable, violent, or emotionally volatile can result in people becoming overly fearful and anxious. This is a scenario that is frequently heard in any discussion of the personality traits of chronic migraineurs.

Learning about the personality traits that are linked to migraines was another "aha" moment that really shook me up. I thought I was reading a description of me since I can best be described as a "perfectionist who has a strong inner critic, who is a serial caretaker, and who is anxious and fearful." My brain was the loser, constantly in a state of fear.

Challenging Life Stressors

I was stunned to learn about the role life stressors, beyond those in childhood, can play in the development and frequency of migraines. Studies find that four out of five of migraineurs believe stress is a major trigger of their migraines. They are not imagining this because research validates this perception.

Life events that are considered "negative" can be highly stressful, such as the death of a spouse, marital separation or divorce, a physical or sexual assault, serious health issues, death of a family member, losing a job, financial problems, or family conflicts. Even events that are considered "positive" can be highly stressful, including pregnancy or birth of a child, marriage, or retirement. Finally, some stressful events can be considered "neutral", such as moving to a new home, beginning or ending school, or changing employment.

In individuals prone to migraines, the more stressful events they are dealing with at one time, the higher the probability that migraines will occur. For example, if someone gets a new job, that is one layer of stress, relocating to a new city to take it is another layer of stress, and, if there is marital conflict over the move, that is a further layer of stress.

Looking back, I recognize a clear pattern in my response to stressful events: give me a new experience and I will have migraines. Triggers included starting high school, college, graduate school, first job, getting married, having children, starting a business, getting divorced, getting married again, and the *coup de grace* for me: retirement.

Key Takeaways from what I Learned about how Chronic Migraines can Develop

What I wrote in the first chapter fits so well here.

> *I began to think maybe, just maybe, the cause of my migraines was not a chronic disease but rather the impact on my neurophysiology of stressors experienced throughout life.*

That sums up an important part of my thinking as I finished exploring this important topic. I also found myself paraphrasing these words from Donna Jackson Nakazawa:

> *Your emotional biography will become your physical biography but it does not have to become your destiny.*

In other words, my emotional biography (childhood stress, highly sensitive make up, personality traits, repressed emotions etc.) had resulted in physical biography (my brain being stressed and the subsequent onset of migraines) but does not have to become destiny (my brain could be healed and my migraines potentially cured).

CHAPTER 3

A New Perspective on Chronic Migraines: The New Neuroscience of Migraine Pain

What next intrigued me about the TMS treatment approach for migraines was the latest brain research which serves as one of its important cornerstones. These studies serve as the foundation for what is referred to as the "*new neuroscience of migraine pain*." I must state that what I learned about this research forever changed how I viewed my migraine pain, and I can't believe my reaction was unique. I must believe that many migraine sufferers could benefit from what I came to understand. Therefore, I'm going to summarize what I found.

Migraine Pain Originates in the Brain

As I began my quest to learn more about the new neuroscience of migraine pain, I was exposed to a concept that was completely foreign to my layman's understanding of pain. It can be summarized in the following phrase by Howard Schubiner, MD, an internationally noted professor of medicine at Michigan State University: *"The reign of pain lies mainly in the brain."* What does he mean by this?

Though the nerves in different parts of the body can send danger signals to the brain, the latest findings in pain science explain that migraine symptoms, pain, nausea, dizziness etc. do not exist until the brain says they do.

This was a concept that was, truthfully, hard for me to swallow or fully understand until I read about the following fascinating example. Many individuals who have limbs amputated still perceive they are having excruciating pain in the limb that is no longer a part of their body. This condition is known as *Phantom Limb Pain*. Just think about this condition for a second. If someone has a limb amputated, how can they feel pain in a body part that is no longer connected? Obviously, this can't be so. There is only one logical answer to this dilemma: the pain signals are not originating from the body part but from the brain.

Migraine Pain is a Danger Signal, but One need not be so Frightened by it

Pain is far and away the number one symptom migraine sufferers report. Close to ninety per cent report having pain when they get a migraine. All pain is a "danger signal" that lets one know that something is amiss in the body. We all know pain's danger signals can be lifesaving, such as when you have a serious physical injury or medical condition like cancer, a heart attack etc.

When migraine symptoms began, like most sufferers, I would be scared, and I was worried that such intense pain was an indicator that my brain was going to be damaged. I have come to learn that fear was not warranted.

Some people with migraines do show changes in their brain known as lesions. Seeing this can be worrisome. Current research simply does not show that such changes in the brain indicate an increased risk of cognitive decline. From what I understand, there is no solid research that having migraines causes long term damage to the brain.

Digesting the implication of these medical findings, I began to think,

> *Perhaps, you don't need to panic, go right to bed and pull the covers over your head when your migraines start. If the pain does not signify damage or danger, then it could be time to try your best to get on with your life instead?*

Pain Experts have Identified a New Category of Pain

Until just the last few years ago pain was broadly classified into two categories: *nociceptive* and *neuropathic.* Just recently, the prestigious *International Association for the Study of Pain* has identified a third category of pain: *nociplastic.* I want to explain why I came to understand the difference between these categories and why they can be potentially so important for chronic migraine sufferers.

Nociceptive pain

This is the pain that most of us are most familiar with. It is pain that results from a process that is taking place in the body. This includes pain from tissue damage like a cut, bruise, or burn. In addition, it can come from inflammation, sprains, pulled muscles, broken bones, or tumors and cancer.

Neuropathic pain

This type of pain is caused by physical damage to the nervous system. Conditions that can damage the nervous system and cause this kind of pain include diabetes, multiple sclerosis, alcoholism, and chemotherapy.

Nociplastic pain

Nociplastic pain is a recently identified category. This is pain that does not have a physical cause that can be identified by diagnostic tests. It is the result of a dysfunction of the pain processing system that produces the sensation of pain without any evidence of physical injury, organ disease, or structural abnormality. Some conditions that fall into this pain category include fibromyalgia, irritable bowel syndrome, many cases of chronic low-back pain, and, most importantly for me, migraines.

The causes of nociplastic pain are still being investigated and aren't fully understood yet, but researchers continue to investigate.

> *Nociplastic pain can be diagnosed because it often originates during times of emotional stress. There is no physical injury or illness. It might be connected with other nociplastic symptoms, and the individual might have experienced physical or emotional adversity during childhood.*

Treatment for nociplastic pain is very different from other types of pain. In general, medications including opioids and non-steroidal anti-inflammatory drugs do not work. Strikingly, treatments that have been shown to be effective in reducing nociplastic pain include patient education and psychological therapies.

Before being exposed to the new neuroscience research, I had never heard about nociplastic pain in any source I had reviewed about migraines or their treatment, and no physician or pain psychologist I saw had ever discussed it or how it can be treated. Learning about this newly recognized category of pain, I began to wonder if all the medications and treatments I had utilized were totally ineffective because they were treating the wrong pain type. Again, it motivated me to look for new treatment answers.

The Power of the Brain to Produce Symptoms

Most laypeople like me underestimate the capacity of the brain to impact physical health. Here are just a few dramatic examples I found.

- The brain can cause individuals to become paralyzed or lose their inability to speak. This is known as a "conversion disorder." Medical tests can demonstrate that there is no nerve or muscle damage, and if the individual gets the proper psychological help, then symptoms can be reversed.
- In a condition known as *Couvade Syndrome*, men whose wives are pregnant can develop the symptoms of pregnancy.
- Medical students frequently get the symptoms of the disorders they have been studying.
- Most astonishingly, there are documented cases of the brain causing death when induced by a voodoo curse, a cruel prank, or a "broken heart."

Since the brains of individuals who are under high levels of emotional stress produce such intense physical symptoms, I had to ask myself the following question: why couldn't it produce the symptoms I was experiencing with my migraines? My answer was that it was as logical a possibility to consider as a biomedical cause.

The Migraine Pain Produced by the Brain is "Real"

To be honest, when I first read about how the brain can create physical symptoms such as migraines, I thought it was "*new age*" nonsense. Little did I understand how the brain functions and the role emotions play in the process influencing how the brain produces such physical changes.

It is commonly recognized that emotions can produce physical changes in the body: someone gets anxious, and they may get nauseous or dizzy or their palms sweat; an individual gets tense and a headache results or they feel a knot in their abdomen; someone gets depressed, and they have no energy. Again, it must be noted that these physical changes are produced by signals from the brain. All these physical symptoms are real; they are not imagined.

I learned that emotions could influence the brain to produce migraine symptoms. Did this mean that they are "all in my head?" In other words, was I simply neurotic, a malingerer, or experiencing a "psychosomatic" condition? I learned the answer, to my relief, was a resounding "NO"! How can I say this with such conviction?

In the depth of my migraines, my neurologist ordered a FMRI brain scan. When she gave me the results, she commented on how the regions of the brain that indicate you're experiencing pain were, in her words, "lit up like a Christmas Tree." I now understand that such a clear diagnostic finding offered conclusive proof that my pain was real, no matter that its origin was my thoughts and feelings and not a physical condition.

The Severity of Migraine Symptoms is the "*Best Guess*" made by the Brain

For all intents and purposes, I learned my migraine pain is my brain's "*best guess*" about what the intensity of my migraine symptoms should be. The brain's responsibility is to integrate scattered signals from a variety of sensory channels, plus information from past experiences, and then produce a sensory experience that it *guesses would be best* to ensure I was *safe* from a danger that the brain perceives.

The brain's "best guess" is not always accurate

Building upon the previous concept, even more important was the next one I was exposed to. Here goes. Our brains can do amazing feats: get man to the moon, cure polio, create the statue of David. Our brains, though, are not infallible, especially when it comes to "guessing" about the severity of the level of the migraine pain one should be experiencing. Here is one classic example to illustrate this point, related to an individual's experience of pain and described in the *British Medical Journal* in 1995.

> *A construction worker fell and landed on a nail that went all the way through his boot. Looking at his boot he was suddenly in excruciating pain and was then rushed to the emergency room where he had to be sedated. When he was finally calm enough, the doctors cut his boot away – and found the nail had miraculously gone between his toes. Seeing that his foot was not harmed, his pain immediately stopped!*

Recognizing that the severity of my migraine symptoms was no more than a "*best guess*" made by my brain and not always accurate was another real eye opener to me. For the first time, I had a glimmer of hope that if this was so, maybe there was something I could do to help my brain make a "*better guess*" that was not so debilitating to me.

Central Sensitization and the Development of Chronic Migraine Pain

My brain's "best guess" was affected by another factor I experienced. As my migraines became more chronic, they were not only getting more frequent but also more severe. This added to my fear and worry. Unfortunately, none of my physicians at the time explained to me the phenomenon that was taking place, and that I was later to learn, is known as "central sensitization."

Central sensitization is a condition of the nervous system that is associated with the development and maintenance of chronic pain. When central sensitization occurs, the brain goes through a process called *wind-up* and gets regulated in a persistent state of high reactivity. This persistent state of reactivity lowers the threshold for what sensations result in pain or other symptoms.

The following analogy illustrates what I realized was the impact central sensitization had on my migraine symptoms.

When I developed central sensitization, my brain began functioning like a defective smoke alarm. Now, a well-functioning smoke alarm is a valuable safety device that warns of danger. But if the alarm becomes so sensitive that it goes off every time you light a candle, it quickly becomes a major annoyance. When my brain became so sensitive, it began constantly sending out alarms when they were not needed.

Central sensitization was playing a significant role in making my migraine pain chronic. With further effort, I was soon to learn about treatment strategies (which will be discussed later) that could enable me to "fix my defective smoke alarm" and reverse the progressive severity of my migraines.

Migraine Symptoms are Significantly Influenced by Thoughts and Feelings

Contrary to what I had previously believed, I came to see that the role my thoughts and feelings played in the severity of my symptoms could not be overstated. This was a profound mind-body connection in my chronic migraine condition. Here are some of the thoughts and feelings that can impact the severity of symptoms.

Paying attention to symptoms makes them feel worse

When my migraines were chronic, I would lie in bed day after day obsessing about my symptoms, constantly monitoring their severity: "*My headache is getting a little worse,*" "*My nausea has been here since I woke up,*" "*Maybe I should try to walk but my dizziness may get worse.*" Little did I realize that constantly thinking about my symptoms was in fact making them much worse. Studies I read clearly made this point, the more I distracted myself from the symptoms the less severe they would become.

Catastrophizing increases severity of symptoms

Along with my migraines becoming chronic came days filled with constant, almost obsessive, scary thoughts: "*The pain and nausea are terrible!*" "*It's never going to get better,*" "*I can't stand it anymore.*" I learned through my research that this extremely negative, fear-filled thinking is what is known as "*catastrophizing.*" It was not helping me, and, in fact, I finally understood it was making my pain worse by constantly sending a signal to my brain that I was in danger.

The Pain Fear Cycle

I eventually realized that my daily catastrophizing resulted in my experiencing what can best be described as the *Pain Fear Cycle*. This phenomenon has three aspects.

1. Migraine pain (or another symptom) begins.
2. The pain (or other symptom) is reacted to with fear, "*Oh no, I can't miss another day of work but I'm too sick to get there,*" "*My head hurts so bad, and my medicine is not helping. What am I going to do?*"
3. Fear then exacerbates the intensity of the symptom which, in turn, keeps the "cycle" going.

The more I catastrophized, the more I was telling my brain that it was in danger. Then, the more my brain got stressed, the more that fueled the intensity of my pain. To put it mildly, my Pain Fear Cycle got out of control and was a major contributor to my daily suffering. I learned this was true for other migraine sufferers I talked with.

The Good News: It is Possible to Change how the Brain Responds to Stress and Reduce or Eliminate Migraines

For many decades, it was thought that by the time one became an adult the brain was unable to change the way it functioned. If one grew up anxious, one was always going to be anxious, if hypersensitive to migraine symptoms, then always hypersensitive. In other words, "*you can't teach an old dog a new trick*." It was enlightening to learn that perspective has been debunked.

Reading about the new research into what is called neuroplasticity taught me that my brain was constantly adapting and rewiring itself.

I came to understand that my brain was like an interconnected power grid with countless roads or *neural pathways* lighting up every time I had a thought or feeling. Some of these roads are well traveled, habitual ways of thinking, feeling, and doing. Every time I was fearful of making a mistake, worried about my health, or pushed down my feelings, I strengthened a road, and it became easier for my brain to travel this pathway.

I also learned that one reason why it is so difficult to change the way I think, feel, and behave is that beliefs and corresponding neural pathways are formed early in life. They have been reinforced and strengthened over time repeatedly. In other words, my brain activity has carved out a deep and well-traveled road. If that road remains and no new roads are built and strengthened, it is very difficult to change my ways, and it is easy to fall back into old patterns.

For me, the most empowering "good news," was that through neuroplasticity new roads can be built. I recognized there were times I changed a bad habit or solved a problem and that carved a new pathway in my brain. I had experienced neuroplasticity firsthand.

I began to think I did not have to continue worrying and catastrophizing or over-responding to every migraine symptom or be stuck in a fear cycle. I began to have hope that there could be an answer to handling my migraines.

The Surprising Benefit of Learning about the New Neuroscience of Pain

As I completed my reading about the new neuroscience of pain, the frequency and severity of my migraines began to improve some. Since the frequency of my migraines did wax and wane somewhat, I did not register any connection whatsoever between the change in my migraines and learning about the new pain science.

I came to realize that my understanding of the new brain science was, in fact, my first step in soothing and healing my brain and building new neural pathways. Let me explain:

I recently was introduced to a new treatment method for pain management known as *Pain Neuroscience Education.* The foundation of this method is to teach chronic pain sufferers about the recent breakthroughs in the science of pain. Studies find that through learning about this new pain science, individuals can change the way they think about pain. This allows them to introduce new ways to respond to painful stimuli, effectively changing their actual experience of pain. This process can help heal the brain and reduce the severity and frequency of migraine episodes.

However, I did not comprehend (at first) that as I was reading about the *New Neuroscience of Pain,* I was creating my own personal *Pain Neuroscience Education* program. I was unconsciously beginning to soothe and heal my brain and nervous system and the arc of my recovery had begun.

STEP TWO OF MY RECOVERY

I Recognized and Accepted the TMS Diagnosis was Right for Me

CHAPTER 4

Accepting A TMS Treatment Approach was Right for Me: Did I Have TMS?

All that I had learned about the new neuroscience of pain and how migraines developed definitely got me thinking that my migraines were a symptom of TMS, but to be fully convinced, I looked into the diagnostic criteria that physicians believe need to be met for someone like me to be diagnosed with the condition. Here is what I understood them to be.

Factors that Increase the Likelihood that TMS is Responsible for Migraines

- A physician has ruled out that there is a structural or physical issue that would explain the migraine symptoms,
- The individual was raised in an emotionally or physically stressful environment,
- The individual meets the criteria for a highly sensitive person,
- The individual has TMS personality traits,
- The individual has or has had other potential TMS symptoms, and
- The individual's migraine symptoms began or worsened during stressful times.

A Physician has Ruled Out that there is a Physical Issue that Would Explain Migraine Symptoms

First off, individuals must rule out a physical issue causing their symptoms, which means they must have a thorough examination by a physician. For most migraine sufferers, that may include having an MRI to make sure there is no structural problem with the brain. In some cases, chronic migraines may be an underlying symptom of another serious condition.

The Individual was Raised in an Emotionally or Physically Stressful Environment

To restate, studies tell us that a stressful or traumatic childhood can be an important factor in the development of migraines. The more emotionally or physically challenging childhood experiences individuals encountered, the higher probability they develop migraines.

One way to begin addressing the reality of the impact of one's childhood experience is to answer the following question, presented to me by Dr David Clarke:

> *If you learned that a child you care about was growing up exactly as you did, how would that make you feel?*

There are further questions that can help someone get a clearer picture as to the level of stress they experienced as a child. Here are some samples adapted from Dr. Howard Schubiner's *Unlearn Your Pain*:

In regards to either parent or caretaker:

- Did you feel loved by them?

- Was their love conditional?
- Were they critical or judgmental?
- Did they have unrealistically high expectations of you?
- Did they abuse alcohol or drugs?
- Did they have mental health issues?
- Were they emotionally neglectful or abusive?
- Were they physically abusive?

Were there particularly stressful or traumatic events in your childhood?

- Death or serious illness of a close relative?
- Marital discord or divorce?
- Financial distress?
- Unstable living situation?
- Incarceration of a parent or parents?
- Severe bullying and teasing by siblings or classmates?
- Physical or sexual abuse?

Reflecting on their answers, the individual feels s/he experienced undue emotional or physical stress during childhood.

The Individual meets the Criteria for being Identified as Highly Sensitive

Again, highly sensitive individuals tend to be more affected by stress and have an increased probability of having migraines that are a result of TMS. The following questionnaire is based upon the work of Elaine Aron, PhD:

- I tend to be very sensitive to pain.
- I have a rich and complex inner life.
- I feel other people's moods affect me. I am conscientious.

- I notice and enjoy delicate or fine scents, tastes, sounds, and works of art.
- When people are uncomfortable in a physical environment, I tend to know what needs to be done to make it more comfortable (like changing the lighting or the seating arrangement).
- I find it unpleasant to have a lot going on at once.
- Being very hungry creates a strong reaction in me, disrupting my concentration or mood.
- I try to avoid violent movies and TV shows.
- When I was a child, my parents or teachers seemed to see me as sensitive or shy.
- I find myself needing to withdraw during busy days, into bed or a darkened room or anyplace where I can have some privacy and relief from stimulation.
- I am easily overwhelmed by things like bright lights, strong smells, coarse fabrics, or loud sirens.
- I startle easily.

It is important to note that although there are as many men as women who are highly sensitive, when taking the test highly sensitive men answer slightly fewer items as true than do highly sensitive women.

Reflecting upon their answers the individual meets the criteria for being a highly sensitive individual.

The Individual has Migraineur Personality Traits

From the experience of TMS practitioners, it is again clear that migraineurs with definite personality characteristics can find this treatment approach highly effective. Here are the questions for individuals to answer in determining if they possess such traits:

Would you describe yourself as:

- Having low self-esteem,
- Being a perfectionist,
- Having overly high expectations of yourself,
- Wanting to be good and/or be liked,
- Being overly conscientious,
- Being hard on yourself,
- Being anxious and fearful,
- Feeling overly responsible for the well-being or feelings of others, and/or
- Difficulty expressing negative emotions?

The Individual has or has had other Potential TMS Symptoms

Individuals whose migraines are the result of a Mind-Body Syndrome often have suffered from other symptoms that medical tests indicate do not have an actual physical cause. The more of these symptoms or conditions that individuals have experienced, the higher the likelihood their migraines could be a product of TMS.

Among these conditions that have been recognized that can be the result of stress:

- Fibromyalgia,
- Tension headaches,
- Neuro muscular pain,
- Temporomandibular joint (TMJ) syndrome,
- Chronic abdominal and pelvic pain syndromes,
- Vulvodynia,
- Piriformis syndrome,
- Repetitive strain injury,
- Foot pain syndromes,

- Myofascial pain syndrome, and
- Chronic back pain.

Autonomic nervous system disorders, including:

- Irritable bowel syndrome,
- Interstitial cystitis (irritable bladder syndrome),
- Postural orthostatic tachycardia syndrome (POTS),
- Inappropriate sinus tachycardia, and
- Reflex sympathetic dystrophy (complex regional pain syndrome).

Other conditions that can occur in patients with Mind-Body Syndrome include:

- Anxiety,
- Depression,
- Obsessive-compulsive disorder,
- Eating disorders, and
- Substance use disorders.

Additional symptoms can include:

- Insomnia,
- Paresthesia (numbness, tingling, burning),
- Tinnitus (ringing in the ears),
- Dizziness,
- Trigeminal Neuralgia,
- Burning chest pain (resembles acid reflux),
- Chronic cough, and
- Chronic hives.

Mind-Body Conditions do <u>not</u> include:

- Cancers,

- Rheumatoid conditions, and
- Infections.

Given your response, do you feel you have had other symptoms or conditions that could be caused by a Mind-Body Syndrome?

Symptoms began or return during Stressful Times

Did the migraine symptoms begin during a time when the individual was under undue stress, and did the migraine symptoms return or worsen during times of stress?

I'm a "Perfect Storm" of TMS Characteristics

I'll never forget as I finished answering all the above questions, rushing to my wife and loudly stating, "I'm a perfect storm of TMS symptoms." It was a classic "OMG" moment for me. No question, no doubt, there could possibly be another answer for the cause of the symptoms that had consumed my life.

Why did I come to this conclusion?

- A physician had ruled out a physical issue that would explain the migraine symptoms? **Yes**
  (Ten physicians that I saw)

- The individual raised in an emotionally or physically stressful environment? **Yes**
  (See previous chapter)

- The individual meets the criteria for a highly sensitive person? **Yes**
  (See previous chapter)

- The individual has TMS personality traits? **Yes**
  (See previous chapter)

- The individual has or has had other potential TMS symptoms? **Yes**
  (Irritable bowel syndrome, anxiety, Tinnitus, foot pain syndrome, insomnia)

- The individual's migraine symptoms began or worsened during stressful times? **Yes**
  (See previous chapter)

It is important to note that many other migraine sufferers I interviewed did not have a "perfect storm" of TMS characteristics such as I did.

I Finally Came to the Conclusion: my Migraines were a Symptom of TMS

To restate, I initially had a great deal of skepticism about the TMS diagnosis, but given all that I had read about neuroscience, how migraines developed, and being a "perfect storm" of TMS characteristics, I "once and for all" believed I had TMS.

Since I could accept the fact that my migraines were a symptom of TMS, the next issue for me was that I did not believe the approach could help me cure them.

CHAPTER 5

ACCEPTING A TMS TREATMENT APPROACH WAS RIGHT FOR ME: BELIEVING IT WILL HELP

Alright, as just stated, I could accept that I had TMS, but could I actually accept such an approach that had seemed so "outside the box" would help with my migraines? In my investigation into this approach, I kept seeing that believing in it and accepting that it could be helpful was an important step in one's recovery. As Dr. Howard Schubiner writes in his classic *Unlearn Your Pain*:

> *"Those people who are unable to accept that their symptoms are due to MBS (TMS), or who do not develop positive expectations of relief, or who are unable to believe that they can make changes in their health and in their lives are the people who are less likely to improve."*

I want to elaborate on his comments. If, for example, individuals have an illness like diabetes, they can manage the illness by watching their glucose numbers and taking insulin shots or medication. They simply do not need to believe in the diagnosis. However, TMS is very different. As I quickly discovered, with believing and acceptance of TMS comes both psychological and physiological changes that are vital to successfully treating the migraines. Here is why.

Believing in the TMS Approach Dramatically Increases the Probability that will it will be Effective with an Individual's Migraines

Medical research dating as far back as the 1980s clearly lays out the case that people who expect or believe they will improve from a treatment are much more likely to do so. Boosting an individual's positive expectations may be a critical tool to enhance their response to treatment. This is particularly relevant with migraines.

Positive beliefs and the placebo effect with migraines

One of the most commonly recognized examples of the impact of positive belief or expectations in medicine is the *placebo effect*. To start with, the placebo effect refers to a favorable response to a medical intervention, pill, procedure, counseling session etc. that doesn't have a measurable physiological effect but still results in a reduction in the individual's symptoms.

> *Until I did my research about TMS treatments, I held the placebo effect in low regard. I derisively thought if people responded to a "suspect" treatment, it was "just the placebo effect"; they had been fooled in some way and their response was inauthentic. Wow, I had a lot to learn.*

It is commonly recognized that an individual's expectations and beliefs are a critical component of the placebo effect. What is not so well understood is that recent research has shown that taking a placebo can actually produce objective changes in the brain's chemistry. A number of studies have found, for example, that the brain releases natural pain-relieving substances called endorphins when people enrolled in pain studies are given placebos.

Now let's get specifically to the placebo effect and the treatment of migraines. I found that its impact on the treatments of migraines is simply astonishing. The placebo effect is most pronounced and relevant when a treatment's success or failure depends largely on the subjective experiences of patients. That's the case with migraine headaches that are defined primarily by the pain they produce. The research backs this up.

Countless studies have found that numerous placebos can help migraine sufferers who have positive belief as to their effectiveness. The most dramatic research comes from a recent Harvard Medical School study. To summarize the findings, migraine sufferers were given either the popular abortive drug Maxalt or a placebo labeled Maxalt to take when a migraine began. When the data was analyzed, participants who took the placebo they believed was Maxalt had the same reduction in pain as those who took the actual prescription drug.

Is TMS treatment simply a placebo?

Some people suggest that TMS treatments are merely a placebo, but this assertion is wrong. The placebo effect demonstrates the power of belief and expectations to healing migraines. The TMS approach is even more powerful since it addresses the cognitive and emotional issues that often are the cause of chronic migraines. As a result, it offers a cure or at least a long-term reduction in the frequency and severity of migraines. The placebo effect tends to be only short term, meaning after a while, the symptoms tend to come back.

The TMS approach is primarily a process of education and psychology; blind faith is simply not involved as many believe is a key to the placebo effect. Patients must decide that the mind-body approach is a logical and reasonable model to treat their migraines because there is challenging work involved. There is no unproven treatment or miraculous intervention with a "healer," only the acquisition of knowledge. It is the knowledge that facilitates healing.

Believing in the TMS Approach Reduces the "Grip of Fear" that Accompanies Believing One has an Incurable Illness

I remember when I was first diagnosed with migraines the tremendous relief I felt. Wow, there really is something wrong with me that can be treated with numerous available medicines. But, to my dismay, the treatments I was prescribed proved ineffective and my migraines worsened.

I will never forget being told by the doctors that were treating me, "unfortunately, I was a migraineur who had a chronic, incurable form of the illness and that the best hope was to try to manage the frequency and severity of the symptoms."

To say the least, that diagnosis was quite frightening. I came to understand how living day in and day out with the stress that comes from believing I had a serious illness resulted in me staying in a constant state of "fight or flight." This flooded my brain with stress hormones that made my symptoms worse. In addition, believing I was a "helpless victim" of my migraines contributed to me feeling disempowered and depressed, which I'm sure did not help my symptoms one bit.

Like the many migraine sufferers I spoke with, the very fact of believing that I had TMS and not some incurable illness produced a dramatic shift in my mood and mindset. Suddenly, I felt the "hope" that there was truly something I could do to help myself. I did not have to rely upon the expertise of another medical practitioner or sit passively by waiting for the next miracle drug. Along with this, when my migraine symptoms did appear, I did not find myself getting so alarmed and sending such dangerous messages to my brain.

My "Roadblocks" to Believing and Accepting the TMS Diagnosis

Like most migraine sufferers who eventually came to accept that the TMS treatment approach was right for them, I had "roadblocks" to this diagnosis that I had to overcome.

Accepting the TMS diagnosis would mean my migraines were my fault

I initially felt there was something "wrong with me" if I believed my migraines were a result of my personality or emotional issues from my past rather than some medical condition.

This belief was significantly reinforced by the comments of a neurologist I had known personally, who derisively stated "*your migraines were a result of your emotional problems from your divorce, and you need to get over it and get on with your life.*" In other words, he told me I needed to get my "sh*t together." By the way, he simply did not know that I was happily married to my second wife at the time and enjoying my life until the migraines became chronic!

This perceived stigma was not unique to me. John Sarno, M.D. in his classic The Divided Mind, *so aptly writes regarding how patients often feel when they are presented with the reality their symptoms may have a psychological component:*

"Negative words like weird, crazy, kooky, and nuts come to mind. 'It's all in your mind' is almost insulting, implying there's something strange or weak about you or that the symptoms are in your imagination. This is most unfortunate since the symptoms are very real and the result of a very physical process."

Learning from medical experts like Dr. Sarno that my migraine symptoms were a real organic process that was occurring in my brain rather than some emotional problem went a long way in helping me overcome some of my resistance to the diagnosis. It definitely helped me accept what I had perceived as such an "outside the box" treatment approach as TMS.

The skepticism of the medical community fuels doubt

As I have previously mentioned, none of my doctors ever asked me about how I dealt with stress from my childhood or my current life. Even when they could not come up with any other treatments to help me, they never once delved into or discussed the role stress and emotions could play in the development of my symptoms. When I even brought up the question of the role they could play in the severity of my symptoms, (other than the misguided neurologist I previously mentioned), they out of hand "*poo pooed*" this as nonsense.

Looking back with disbelief, even when they were at a loss for what treatment to recommend, they kept reiterating that my migraines had a physical and not emotional cause, period. I now recognize my well trained and well-meaning physicians came to this perspective because:

> *Their training and modes of treatment focus on healing symptoms generated by physical disorders in the body. They are, therefore, understandably loath to consider another diagnosis, particularly one that has a mind-body origin.*

The more I accepted this point of view, the easier it became to believe in a new diagnosis for my migraines.

How I Came to Believing that TMS Would Work for Me

I became aware that believing and acceptance is a process not a single event and that everyone's process is different. Some simply read a book, talk to a friend, or consult a medical practitioner and buy in 100%. Others can take years to finally accept that TMS is the answer for them. My experience was somewhere in between and here are the critical steps of my process.

Desperation fueled my openness to the approach

To be perfectly honest, I doubt if I would have even begun to believe in the TMS approach, which was so outside the box for me, if I had not tried so many other mainstream treatments. I simply did not know where else to turn for a cure. In my state of mind, I was desperate for help.

Hearing the testimonials from migraine sufferers

My desperation even made me open to look at the ad for the Curable app. What actually motivated me to begin to use it were the videos and podcasts of migraine sufferers that it contained. They discussed how they had utilized a TMS approach to recover. To my disbelief, I was seeing and hearing individuals describing how changing their thoughts and feelings and dealing with the challenges they faced in the past enabled them to cure their migraines. More than anything, I was stunned by the fact that they sounded both "believable and convincing" even though they were talking about a healing approach that "flew in the face" of anything I had ever heard of for my migraines.

The evidence-based research foundation of the approach

The Curable app was the catalyst to look into the science behind the TMS approach. Given traditional biomedical based treatments had always been the foundation of my approach to dealing with my health, I had never been a fan of "alternative" medical treatments. Thus, when I initially looked into the TMS approach, I was doubtful that it would be of any help for me.

What kept piquing my interest in the TMS approach was the medical research that was such an integral foundation to the model. Learning about the studies behind the new neuroscience of pain and how stress, emotions, and trauma can predispose one to migraines was mind-boggling. I decided this might be something that could help me.

My TMS characteristics

Recognizing that I was a "perfect storm" of TMS characteristics took me far along the process of accepting that this approach was right for me, but there was still a major question hanging out there: would the treatment strategies work for me?

A physician validated my TMS diagnosis

A major turning point was being lucky enough to see noted TMS physician Dr. David Schechter. After all the MD's I had seen, I never had one who was so probing in his questions about the stress I experienced in my childhood, my personality traits, and how I responded to stress. I will never forget when he finished his exam, he looked at me and simply said, "*your migraines are a symptom of what is known as TMS.*" Even though I had thought this could be so, hearing from a physician of his stature definitely carried more weight for me than anything else. I was finally convinced and ready to use the treatment approach to recover.

STEP THREE OF MY RECOVERY

I Learned How to Soothe and Heal My Brain and Nervous System

CHAPTER 6

I Learned how to Soothe and Heal My Brain and Nervous System: TMS Treatment Strategies that helped My Recovery

Through all my efforts to learn about TMS and how it could help my migraines, I came to the following insights:

- Traditional biomedical treatments simply were not useful to healing my migraines. I no longer had to be a subservient follower of the treatment plans of the medical professionals; I could actually "take charge" of the treatment of my migraines.
- I had examined the science on how chronic stress and trauma could impact the development of my migraines. It was vital for me to remember that the adversity that I faced simply did not determine who I am or can be. The popular phrase "*neither my biography nor biology is my destiny*" had a whole new empowering meaning for me!
- I must keep in mind that neuroscience has now learned that the amazingly neuroplastic brain is capable of incredible changes once appropriate interventions are used.

Bottom line: By soothing and healing my nervous system, I could recover from my migraines!

Empowered by these insights, "*I marched forth on my hero's journey to reclaim my life from migraines.*" (Please excuse the dramatic language but that is how I felt!) More accurately, I utilized the TMS approach I had learned to enable me to soothe and heal my nervous system. Through my understanding of the TMS approach, for the first time I felt "lit up and on fire" and empowered to make a difference in the course of my recovery. What follows is a description of how my efforts enabled me to recover once and for all.

The most important tool that enabled me to "take charge" was the use of the TMS treatment strategies I had been introduced to through my exploration. I want to share those that I found the most useful in my effort to reclaim my life. I should emphasize that the strategies that worked for me were often not the ones that helped other migraine sufferers, and the ones that helped some of them did not always work for me. There simply is no "step-by-step" or "one size fits all" treatment plan to follow.

Thinking Psychologically not Physically

When I initiated my use of a variety of TMS treatment strategies, to my delight the use of one paid off rapidly. It all began on an ordinary day when I woke up with my usual migraine symptoms. It just so happened that on this day I had scheduled a photography lesson. Though I was anxious about the stress I might experience going to it, I still knew I would hate to miss it. As per usual, my fear kicked in and I soon thought "*you had better get back to bed so your pain and dizziness does not get really bad.*" Lucky for me, I had just read about a strategy designed to stop the brain from going into a habitual fear response when symptoms begin known as *Think Psychologically not Physically*.

The cornerstone of this strategy is as follows: when migraine symptoms begin, rather than thinking about the physical cause, think about the cause that could be psychological. To better understand how I utilized this treatment strategy, let me explain what transpired on the aforementioned day.

As my fear began to build, I started an inner dialog. I said to myself, "*you are not sick, your body is OK, there is no physical cause of your migraine symptoms.*" I then took a couple of deep breaths, closed my eyes, and asked myself, "*what stressor is going on today that could be causing my migraine?*" After thinking for a minute, a response came into my head, "*I'm scared to drive to my photography lesson. I may get really sick there and have trouble getting home.*" After taking a few more deep breaths, I said to myself, "*you'll be OK, you are just scared. Worst case scenario, you can either have your wife come to get you or you can Uber home and get your car later.*"

With trepidation, I decided to give it a go. I must admit that I was very nervous driving to the lesson since I still felt "migraine lousy." But as I got engaged with my tutor, my symptoms began to diminish, and by the end of the session, my migraine was absolutely gone! I was stunned, and I remember thinking to myself "*OMG! This TMS approach is the 'real deal' and it really looks like it can help cure my migraines!*"

What had happened? By thinking psychologically and not physically, I was retraining my brain that there is nothing physically wrong with my body and that the migraine had a psychological cause i.e. stress. I saw for the first time that I didn't have to stop my life when I got symptoms because, in most cases, I will be able to just "power through." I will not get sicker but, in actuality, I will end up feeling better! Such an insight helped further the process of soothing and healing my brain which I now knew was, without a doubt, the key to my recovery.

I Am Safe

Another strategy I found incredibly useful when fear raised its dark brooding head was what is known as *I Am Safe*. I used this strategy both when I began to go into fear surrounding my migraine symptoms and throughout the day when I was impacted by the stress of the day.

As I mentioned before, whenever I got a migraine, my neural pathways of fear were activated, and I found myself entering another "pain fear cycle." This cycle describes how pain sensations stimulated my feelings of fear which, in turn, resulted in my experience of pain getting worse and on and on. This cycle unfortunately kept sending danger signals to my brain which I now understand helped keep the migraines coming. Given what I had learned, I was well aware that having migraine symptoms did not mean I was in danger; they were just physical symptoms that I did not have to fear like I had learned to in the past. The antidote for the fear, as well as the key to soothing my brain, was to send it one clear and unequivocal message: "*I am safe.*"

When I experienced my fearful thoughts beginning to cascade down: "Oh no I'm going to be so sick again" - "not another migraine so soon"- "my day may be ruined", I sat down, closed my eyes, took a few deep breaths and began to chant to myself "I am safe, I am safe, I am safe." Sometimes I would add a message such as, "nothing to fear, you're going to be OK!"

I Am Safe became my "safety blanket" at other stressful times during the day as well. When I found myself worrying about everyday issues, be it money or relationships or work, and my worry bone began to kick in catastrophizing about how bad things could be, I would again chant to myself: *I Am Safe.*

Honestly, when I initially tried chanting the *I Am Safe* mantra, I did not find much relief. But as it became the daily mantra of my TMS practice, it was soon a priceless tool that I relied upon. I soon grasped that the consistent use of this practice was enabling me to build new neural pathways that aiding in healing my nervous system in times of stress.

Mindful Meditation

Being a highly sensitive person whose brain had been in a constant state of fight-flight since I was a child, I needed an antidote to the fear, worry, and anxiety that became my frequent companion as my migraines became chronic. Before I began using the TMS approach, I had used mindful meditation for my migraines with no success at all. I had no interest in trying it again until I read the research on how effective it can be.

Recent brain studies tell us that through the use of mindfulness techniques one can actually change the neural pathways in the brain. Of great importance for migraine sufferers is that through the use of meditation, the amygdala, or the part of the brain important to the response to emotional stress, can be significantly calmed.

A real eye opener for me was the medical research on how mindful meditation can improve migraine symptoms. In a 2014 study, migraineurs who used mindfulness meditation for 30 minutes a day over a two-month period reported a dramatic reduction in both the frequency and the severity of their migraines. In another recent study, researchers found that migraine sufferers who meditated on a regular basis for several months reported migraine symptoms were down 28-percent, anxiety was down 44-percent, and depression decreased by 34-percent.

Of utmost importance to me was understanding why my attempts to use mindfulness meditation did not work when I tried it the first time. Believing I had an incurable illness resulted in my being in a state of low-level fear and worry which was a significant stressor for my brain and nervous system. The fear that results from such a belief can blunt much of the benefit of meditation. As I came to accept that I did not have an incurable illness and my brain was not as stressed, my meditation practice produced the results I had hoped it would. My mindfulness meditation practice became a backbone of my daily efforts to heal my brain and recover.

Exercise

Regular exercise became a major challenge for me as my migraines worsened. I either felt too lousy to try, or, when I felt better, I was afraid if I did too much my migraines would become worse. Two factors convinced me to increase my exercise: learning about the research on the positive impact it can have on migraine symptoms and accepting I did not have a physical illness that would worsen if I exercised.

Recent studies I found showed how exercise can help manage the symptoms of migraine in a few different ways. Exercise releases endorphins, which are the body's natural painkillers. Endorphins also induce positive feelings and a sense of well-being which can be especially beneficial for migraine sufferers. Additionally, exercise can improve sleep and lower stress, which are both common migraine triggers.

Finally, studies show that regular exercise can reduce both the frequency and severity of migraine symptoms. One study indicated exercise was as helpful as one of the leading preventative medications.

Believing I was sick was a major detriment to my exercising. Given that a common symptom of my migraines along with the pain, nausea, and cognitive fog was vertigo, I was afraid to walk (my go-to mode of exercise) because I became quite dizzy whenever I tried to do so. As my migraines began to improve, I considered upping the length of my walks, but the fear of getting dizzy, falling, or not being able to get home was still my master.

That was until my wife stepped in with her words of wisdom. One day when I was still in the grip of fear around walking, she asked me the following question: "*you have been dizzy on and off for years, have you ever fallen or been unable to get home?*" I thought for a moment and had to answer "*no.*" She responded, "*you're right, so why do you still need to worry so much?*" I immediately recognized this worry was just another habitual fear response that resulted from me believing I had a physical illness.

Thus, I built walks into my daily treatment routine. Was it easy at first? Absolutely not! On my walks I often got quite dizzy and scared. The antidote was to constantly reassure myself "*I am safe, nothing bad is going to happen to me, I'm not going to fall, I'll make it home OK, I am safe.*" Bless this mantra. It was a life saver for me on more walks than I want to admit.

Expressive Writing

Like many migraine sufferers, I had difficulty expressing feelings, especially those that were threatening or uncomfortable. These feelings came from my current circumstances and those from my past, especially childhood. An effective technique for many migraine sufferers with this issue is *expressive writing*.

My process was to allow 10-20 minutes to write in a quiet location where I would not be interrupted. I would write either when I began to get migraine symptoms or about once a day. I would simply write about what I was feeling at the time. I would not censor any thought or feeling no matter how raw and ugly it might be. I let it all hang out on the page. Finally, I made sure no one ever saw the raw emotion I spewed on the page.

The goal of expressive writing is to uncover repressed feelings and reframe them in a manner that could help my brain and body heal. It had the potential to help me better regulate my emotions and break free from the endless mental cycle of brooding and rumination that often accompanied my migraine symptoms.

Many migraineurs report that through writing, they got in touch with stressful or traumatic events from their past and gained insight into how their feelings about these events were contributing to their emotional hypersensitivity. As they privately wrote about these past difficult experiences, they found they were more able to talk with others about them. The result was feeling enabled to reach out for social, or therapeutic support that could aid their recovery.

I found expressive writing to be challenging. As I used it more and more, I increasingly ended up writing about subjects that brought up feelings from my childhood that were so painful I simply could not continue. But expressive writing did open the door for me to seek psychotherapy from a therapist who had expertise in the TMS approach.

Key Insights that Helped Guide my Use of TMS Treatment Strategies

Taking charge of my recovery and using TMS treatment strategies, though life changing, was no "walk in the park." As I went through the healing process, I gained numerous key insights that would serve as valuable guideposts as I navigated the twists and turns of my recovery.

I should not compare my recovery to that of anyone else

Being the perfectionist I am, I jumped in with both feet into the use of the TMS approach. I was going to be the "poster child" of how to recover from migraines. Then, I heard about someone who read a book, used the Curable App, or saw a TMS specialist and stated their migraines ended overnight. It was a real "bummer" for me. I would find myself ruminating, *"if they could get rid of their migraines like that, why can't I?"* Believing I "should" recover in a certain amount of time because someone else was able to just added more stress to my brain and might have slowed my recovery. For various reasons, some people's migraine symptoms improve within days or weeks but others may take months or longer. Recovery is not a race or contest. Everyone's recovery journey is unique!

The TMS approach is not a "Quick Fix Pill"

Having felt like I had lost my life to migraines for so many years, I was desperate for a cure. Even though my migraines were dramatically improving, having even one a month was too many for me. I was soon beating myself up for not healing fast enough. I got "down in the dumps" whenever I had even a minor setback. I became an insufferable taskmaster, trying to drive myself to a rapid recovery. It obviously did not work.

I never reached a place of equanimity until I grasped that the TMS approach was not going to be a "Quick Fix Pill" that would heal me. As effective as the TMS process can be, I needed to accept that it would take time and effort on my part. Eventually, giving in to the process lowered my stress level and sped up my improvement.

The path of my recovery will not be a straight line upward

Again, being a perfectionist, I magically believed that if I did everything right, I would never have any setbacks in the arc of my recovery. This, I learned the hard way, was ridiculous.

To my dismay, after a month or so of using the TMS strategies the path of my recovery turned precipitously downward. I was devastated until I was able to understand the important role it played in my healing.

First, setbacks are a normal part of the TMS healing process. They are necessary learning opportunities to grasp how to respond better to stressful events. I began to see that the path of my recovery was going to be fluid and that I needed to "ride the waves" as they came. It aided my healing to come to the process with as much equanimity as I could muster instead of with nothing but unrealistic expectations.

Acceptance of my migraines

As strange as it might sound, another insight that helped reduce the stress on my brain was learning to accept that I did have migraines. That needs some explanation.

Day in and day out, I lived in a constant cycle of hope and disappointment based upon whether or not I had a migraine. On days I did not have a migraine,

I would hope beyond hope that they would not return only to have crushing disappointment when they did. This attitude that my well-being was dependent upon how bad my migraine symptoms were was feeding the "stressor beast" that was wearing out my brain. To tame this beast, I had to change my response to my symptoms and take away their power to control my life. I needed to reach the point where:

A good day is not measured by the severity of my migraines, but by how little I cared about them and/or let them stop my day!

The surprising answer, as I finally came to learn, was "*acceptance of what is so - I had migraines.*" I was not able to eliminate my migraines. Acceptance meant that when I got a migraine, no matter how hard this may seem, that it was in my best interest simply to acknowledge it was there.

This contrasted with my habitual response of catastrophizing or judging it as something I did not want. Acceptance did not mean living in resignation that they would never improve. Acceptance meant I needed to do my best to allow my thoughts and feelings around the migraine to just be there.

Let me elaborate on this concept. It became clear to me that whenever I got a migraine, I tried to avoid the feelings of emotional upset that accompanied them. This obviously seemed very sensible because the sensations were very unpleasant. I tried to ignore them, distract myself, or go so far as turning to strong pain medication to numb the discomfort. This avoidance at times worked in the immediate short term, but before long, avoidance failed me. Why? There is a classic saying, "what you resist persists." What the science tells us is that the more you try to resist your negative feelings, the stronger they unfortunately become.

What I learned was hard for me to grasp at first, but it was another building block for my recovery. In the short term, my goal was to recognize that there might be nothing I could do to prevent my migraines from coming on. More important was to change the way I responded to them when they did. I eventually learned that, through acceptance, this was difficult but possible.

I needed to find the "sweet spot" of my recovery efforts

I soon saw that I had to find and maintain a "sweet spot" in my recovery efforts. Throughout my life, I felt I had to work harder than others to achieve my goals. I brought that same, hard driving perspective to my healing. I would try to "binge heal," hoping that if I "obsessively" consumed healing content, meditated, exercised, used expressive writing etc. I would heal quicker, but this did not work! I would stop their use because I got burned out from trying so hard. I finally had to acknowledge that more effort does not always equal more progress.

I eventually found my "sweet spot." I made sure to use the treatment strategies that worked for me just enough to ensure I was keeping the path of my recovery going in a positive direction without finding myself so consumed with effort that I ended up burned out.

I was Beginning to get my Life Back

As the days and weeks of the TMS strategies progressed, the frequency and severity of my migraine symptoms began to decrease. I was relieved and grateful that I was no longer in bed almost daily with migraine symptoms. It is important that I note the following:

I still did frequently get migraine symptoms, but my response to them was radically different than before. No longer did I catastrophize when I began to feel dizzy or experience pain. I was learning to soothe and calm my brain rather than feeding it a strong dose of fear.

As a result, I was amazed to find my old life slowly returning. Though my migraines did limit my activities once or twice a week, I was again able to go on long walks, handle business affairs, keep most social engagements, and spend quality time with my children, grandchildren, and, most importantly, my wife.

The biggest change for me was that my life was not consumed with worrying about when I would be getting my next migraine, or, if I had one, how bad it would get. I felt like I was getting my life back.

CHAPTER 7

I LEARNED HOW TO SOOTHE AND HEAL MY NERVOUS SYSTEM: TMS BASED PSYCHOTHERAPY ENABLED ME TO FINALLY RECLAIM MY LIFE

As much as my migraines had improved, there was still a dark cloud hanging over my head. When I was using expressive writing, I kept getting in touch with a frightening darkness that lived in me. This darkness resulted in constantly feeling there was something "wrong" with me. I believed in some inexplicable way these frightening feelings played a major role in my getting migraines. Further, as my migraines kept improving, I found myself getting more anxious that unless I dealt with these feelings, I would likely get some other ailment or regress in the future.

As a result, I felt that if I was going to further the process of soothing and healing my brain and nervous system, I needed the help of a professional therapist who had experience treating TMS clients.

My search for the right therapist was challenging. I ended up spending much time and money and did not get the help I needed from therapists who did not understand how to treat TMS. After much searching, I was finally blessed to find Derek Sapico, LMFT at the *Pain Psychology Center*. He had a tremendous amount of training and experience in working with individuals who had TMS issues. By working with him, I came to much better understand the issues that produced my migraines and additional strategies to help overcome them.

I had Profound Insights on the role Childhood Stress had on my Physical and Emotional Health

Derek helped me gain profound insights related to my early years.

First, looking back, it was clear my mother had serious emotional problems from the time I was an infant. She was anxious, depressed and emotionally cold; I have no memories of her ever hugging me, complimenting me, or saying she loved me.

I thought I understood how my mother's issues affected me, but, truthfully, I had no conception of the severe impact the stress I lived through had on my psyche and nervous system. Though I did not suffer big "T" trauma, my therapist explained that my upbringing resulted in my experiencing a form of "*emotional death by a thousand cuts.*"

As a result, from a young age anxiety and fear have been a major challenge for me. This, combined with the fact I've been the victim of self-loathing, haunted with the belief that there was something wrong with me, and the fear that if I got too stressed I could end up "crazy" like my mother. I was astonished to see that all of these issues were a direct outgrowth of the impact my childhood stress had on my developing brain and nervous system.

The second insight was the most profound for my migraines. After much help from Derek, I came to the following hard to believe conclusion.

My migraines were an attempt by my brain to protect me from the darkness that was so frightening to me.

Here is how he explained this to me. As a result of the stress and trauma of my childhood, I had a deep, dark belief that I was a worthless, damaged individual who was unlovable. During my adult years, my perfectionist, professional efforts resulted in my achieving tremendous personal and professional recognition that helped me repress the dark feelings that lingered inside me. I came to believe if I could achieve such professional success, maybe I did have some redeeming value after all.

Then the bottom fell out for me: I retired. Left without the safety net of my professional identity, the darkness began to raise its frightening head and overwhelm me. I didn't know how to face life without my professional identity. Psychically, dealing with those feelings was more than I could handle at the time. I was terrified that I might have a breakdown if I couldn't get them pushed down again.

Thus, in an effort to distract me from devastating psychic pain, my brain produced migraines. If I had a migraine, I could go to bed and no one would expect me to get out and be in the real world, meaning my feelings of inadequacy and self-loathing would not overwhelm me.

My migraines could become a new "safety blanket" to keep the darkness away.

Was this hard to accept? You better believe it. Through the work with my therapist, I was able to go into the "dark room" where my fears lived and begin to shine a light on them. Through this process, for the first time in my life I was able to face the fear, sadness, self-loathing, and rage that was at its core. I would talk to that scared little boy who lived within me. I spent much time letting him know he was "safe" and he could finally come out of the darkness where he had dwelled for so long and into the light of life.

As I dealt with the dark feelings, I was grateful to find my migraines rapidly diminishing. I must admit I was stunned, but this was no coincidence. Hard as it was to accept, my brain was using migraines to protect me from the emotional breakdown that I feared. But, when the stress of repressing my feelings receded, my brain calmed down. As it calmed, so did the need to protect me, and my migraines let up.

I Needed to Stop my Emotional Self Abuse

Another residue from childhood was self-loathing that I carried deep inside my psyche. This self-loathing played out in the emotional self-abuse that was a constant in my inner dialog. This inner dialog was a ceaseless negative voice in my head that was stressing my brain by doing the following.

Self-criticism:

Constantly putting me down: "*You can't do anything right," "You're just unlovable" or "Why can't you just do better dealing with your migraines?"*

Undue pressure

Putting myself under undue pressure: *"You're not trying hard enough to get better," "You don't spend enough time with your family," or "You need to do better."*

Fear and worry

Being constantly fearful and or worried: *"I'm afraid my migraines could get worse," "I'm scared I won't know what to do with myself when I retire,"* or *"So worried about my finances."*

The harmful impact of emotional self-abuse

The residue of believing there was something wrong with me needed to be addressed. I never understood the role emotional self-abuse had on my health, especially my migraines. The following analogy drove the point home.

Everyone's brain works much like a computer. An individual's self-talk and beliefs are in many ways like the software program their brain runs. One's brain and body are significantly influenced by the quality of one's inner dialog. Thoughts and judgements are like a computer code which sends instructions every millisecond to the nervous system in ways that have a powerful impact on a person's overall sense of well-being.

> *Of most importance, an individual's self-talk can either increase the level of stress, anxiety, and feelings of being overwhelmed or ease the level of stress and help create a sense of inner well-being.*

One way of thinking about this is to imagine that your self-talk is like a radio station that is playing all the time in the background. Being self-abusive resembles tuning into the "Abuse Channel" that is constantly sending negative self-talk messages. Over time, that will keep you in a state of low-grade fight-flight-freeze. This is a constant stressor on the brain.

Practice self-compassion

While in therapy, I learned that if I was going to change the "channel" in my head from abusive to one that was soothing to my brain, I needed to practice self-compassion. This therapeutic approach is based upon the ground-breaking research of Kristin Kneff, PhD.

In a nutshell, self-compassion entails being loving and understanding towards yourself when you suffer, fail, or feel inadequate rather than ignoring your pain or flagellating yourself with self-criticism or harsh judgment.

Perhaps most importantly, having self-compassion means that you honor and accept your humanity. Life will not always go the way you want. You will encounter frustrations, losses will occur, you will make mistakes, bump up against limitations, and fall short of your ideals. This is the human condition, a reality shared by all of us.

When this reality is denied or struggled against, suffering increases in the form of stress, frustration, and self-criticism. When this reality is accepted with sympathy and kindness, greater emotional equanimity can be found and the level of stress experienced by the brain reduced.

How I learned to practice self-compassion

A cornerstone of self-compassion is the ability to respond to myself like a friend. If I was self-critical or judgmental because I "screwed up," I learned to stop and ask myself the following question: *if a good friend made the same mistake or had the same shortcoming, how would I respond?* I would be much more compassionate and understanding. I then would try to respond to myself the same way.

Developing self-compassion was challenging. My self-critical, judgmental inner voice was such a part of me that there were many times I was not aware of how it was beating me up. It took much practice to recognize when this was occurring and how poorly it made me feel.

In addition, at times I had trouble responding to myself as a compassionate friend. A tool I found very helpful was to sit down and write myself a letter from the perspective of this friend. Putting my thoughts on paper was a game changer for getting in touch with the self-compassion I needed to further my healing.

The greatest gift I received from self-compassion was, for the first time in my life, actually feeling self-love. I no longer felt I was worthless or unlovable. Did I have faults and shortcomings? Absolutely! Was I still a decent person deserving of love? Again, absolutely! I'm so very grateful to learn to have compassion for myself.

AFTERWORD

As I write this, I can stand up and exclaim to all; "I have my life back!" Do I still occasionally get migraine symptoms? Yes. Do I still get anxious? Yes. Does it affect the quality of my life? Absolutely not!

Of much greater importance to my sense of equanimity and happiness are the following:

For the first time in my life, I have come to understand how the adversity of my childhood and other life stressors have impacted my mental and physical health. My biology truly does not have to become my destiny. No longer do I have to be a victim of my past circumstances. It is possible for me to heal and reboot my brain. Even though my nervous system has been set on a high reactive mode for decades, I have been able to dial it down.

If I only knew when I was younger what I know now, I'm confident I would not have spent years in bed suffering with migraines.

I have begun to make a life-affirming mental shift. No longer do I feel my life is consumed and driven by dark negative thoughts and feelings; I have found the courage to confidently put them in their rightful place, and allow positive uplifting ones to guide me. As a result, I am able to respond to life's challenges in a more gratifying manner.

I have finally come to understand that healing is about more than fixing what was wrong with me.

At last, I have begun to feel safe and at home in my mind and body. I'm continuously more able to focus on what gives me a deeper sense of relaxation, safety and calm, and rest my attention there. I'm able to increase my ability to flourish even in difficult times.

In conclusion, I know this may sound crazy, but I have come to see that my migraines were in a strange way a gift trying to teach me a lesson I could not learn in any other way. They were "thoughtful messengers" letting me know that the way I was dealing with my emotions and stressors was both harmful and possibly life threatening. By putting in the work to finally listen to what they wanted to teach me, I can state for all to hear:

I feel a level of peace the likes of which I had never before dreamt I could feel. I can honestly state, I have reclaimed a better life than I ever thought possible!

RESOURCES THAT I FOUND USEFUL FOR MY RECOVERY

APPS

Curable

BOOKS

They Can't Find Anything Wrong: David Clarke, MD

The Way Out: Alan Gordon and Alon Ziv

Back in Control: David Hanscom, MD

The Body Keeps Score: Brain, Mind, and Body in the Healing of Trauma: Bessel van der Kolk

Childhood Disrupted: How Your Biography Becomes Your Biology, and How You Can Heal: Donna Jackson Nakazawa

The Mind-Body Prescription: John Sarno, MD

Healing Back Pain: John Sarno, MD

Think Away Your Pain: David Schechter, MD

Unlearn Your Pain: Howard Schubiner, MD

Radical Self-Compassion: Tara Brach

Self-Compassion: The Proven Power of Being Kind to Yourself: Kristen Neff PhD

TMS HEALTHCARE PRACTITIONERS

Psychophysiological Disorder Association Directory of Healthcare Practitioners:
https://www.ppdassociation.org//directory

PODCASTS

Like Mind Like Body with Curable

Tell Me about your Pain with Alan Gordon

The Cure for Chronic Pain with Nicole Sachs

FACEBOOK GROUPS

Curable

Curable Community

Tell Me About Your Pain Community

TMS The Mind-Body Syndrome

John Sarno Support Group

WEBSITES

Psychophysiological Disorder Association:
www.ppdassocation.org

TMS wiki:
www.tmswiki.org

Curable Health:
www.curablehealth.com

Self-Compassion:
www.Self-Compassion.org

DOCUMENTARIES

This Might Hurt
https://www.thismighthurtfilm.com/buy-the-film

All the Rage: Saved by Sarno
https://www.amazon.com/All-Rage-Saved-Sarno-John/dp/B07NYCXH7V/ref=sr_1_1?dchild=1&keywords=saved+by+sarno&qid=1615576160&sr=8-1

Pain Brain
https://painbrainfilm.com/

Ted Talk: *Is there scientific proof we can heal ourselves?* Lissa Rankin, MD
https://www.youtube.com/watch?v=LWQfe__fNbs

ACKNOWLEDGEMENTS

Before I finish, I must take a brief minute to acknowledge the individuals without whose help and support this memoir would not have been possible.

Dr. John Sarno, the father of the TMS treatment model. The Curable Health team which developed the app that began my journey. Drs. David Schechter, David Clarke, Howard Schubiner, and John Stracks who all taught me much about how to use the TMS treatment approach with my migraines. Derick Sepico, LMFT, the best psychotherapist I have ever had.

Kristen and Maira from PRESStinely for being as good a publishing team I have ever worked with. Thanks for making this book look as good as it does.

Josh and Nicole, your love and support was so important to me when I was struggling with my migraines. Finally, to Barbie, your care, love and optimism, enabled me to get through the darkest time of my life.

www.ingramcontent.com/pod-product-compliance
Ingram Content Group UK Ltd.
Pitfield, Milton Keynes, MK11 3LW, UK
UKHW021411020425
5280UKWH00042B/418

9 798986 275802